Eat Right

Drink Pure

Be Well

A Comprehensive Guide to
Healthy Drinking and Eating

Dr. Myles Watson Collins

Foreword

In today's busy world, what we eat matters more than ever. The food choices we make affect not only our health but also the health of our planet. Understanding how our diet impacts our lives and the environment is crucial.

"Eat Right, Drink Pure, Be Well: A Comprehensive Guide to Healthy Drinking and Eating" by Dr. Myles Watson Collins is an important book that helps us understand the link between food and health. Dr. Collins, with his years of research and experience, offers practical advice on how to make better food choices that can improve our health and benefit the environment.

Good nutrition is key to staying healthy. A balanced diet with the right nutrients can prevent diseases, boost our immune system, and improve our overall well-being. On the other hand, poor eating habits can lead to problems like obesity, diabetes, heart disease, and cancer. This book provides simple steps to help us eat healthier and live better lives.

Our food choices also impact the planet. How food is grown, transported, and consumed affects the environment. By choosing sustainable, plant-based, and local foods, we can reduce our environmental footprint and help create a more sustainable food system. Dr. Collins explains how making these choices is good for both our health and the planet.

This book is a helpful guide full of clear, practical advice. Dr. Collins uses the latest research to clear up common myths about diet and health. He emphasizes the importance of whole foods, balanced meals, and mindful eating, offering a realistic approach to nutrition.

As you read "Eat Right, Drink Pure, Be Well," I hope you feel inspired to make healthier food choices. This book can help you nourish your body, improve your mind, and protect our planet. Together, we can create a healthier, more sustainable future.

Connie Prather, MD, MPH
Director of Public Health Initiatives
Gut Health Institute, Peace-World General Hospital

About the Author

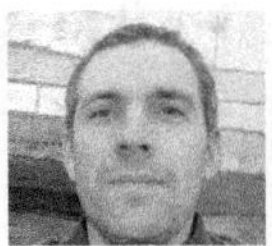 Dr. Myles Watson Collins is a leading nutritionist and health expert with over 20 years of experience in the field. He holds a Ph.D. in Nutrition from Harvard University and is a certified dietitian. Dr. Collins has dedicated his career to studying the impact of diet on health and disease prevention.

In addition to his work at the hospital, Dr. Collins also runs the Revitalize Wellness Center, a premier wellness facility located in the heart of New York City, where he offers personalized nutrition and wellness plans, fitness programs, and stress management to help individuals achieve optimal health through natural and science-backed methods. Dr. Collins and his dedicated team work tirelessly to help individuals achieve their health goals and improve their quality of life.

Dr. Collins is an avid writer and has contributed numerous articles to prestigious newspapers and journals, including The New York Times, The Washington Post, Health Journal, and Nutrition Science Review.

His research focuses on the benefits of whole foods, the role of macronutrients and micronutrients in health, and the prevention of chronic diseases through diet.

In addition to his research, Dr. Collins has worked with various health organizations to develop nutrition guidelines and educational materials. He is passionate about making nutrition information accessible and practical for everyone.

Dr. Collins's dedication to improving public health through nutrition education has earned him numerous awards and recognition. He continues to inspire and educate others on the importance of healthy eating and lifestyle choices.

In addition to his professional accomplishments, Dr. Collins is an avid cyclist and enjoys exploring the scenic routes of New York. He is also a passionate cook, often experimenting with new healthy recipes that he shares with his clients and followers. He enjoys gardening, which he finds to be a relaxing and rewarding hobby as well. He believes that growing his own vegetables not only supports his family's health but also deepens his connection with nature.

Dr. Collins lives in Brooklyn, New York, with his wife, Kathleen, and their three children, Rebecca, Deborah, and James. His family is his greatest source of inspiration and support. Dr. Collins' commitment to his family and his community is reflected in his dedication to promoting healthy living and wellness for all.

Dr. Collins's passion for Optimal health extends beyond his professional and writing endeavors. He frequently speaks at conferences and seminars, sharing his knowledge and inspiring others to take charge of their health through better nutrition, diet, and lifestyle choices.

Contents

Introduction

Rose had always struggled with her health. From her early twenties, she battled constant fatigue, digestive issues, and fluctuating weight. Despite trying various diets and fitness routines, nothing seemed to work. She felt trapped in a cycle of temporary solutions and persistent problems. Rose's journey to better health was filled with frustration, until she discovered the power of eating right and drinking pure.

Rose's turning point came during a visit to a new doctor who suggested she try a grain-free, whole foods diet. Skeptical at first, Rose decided to give it a shot. She replaced processed foods with fresh vegetables, fruits, lean proteins, and healthy fats. She also cut out sugary drinks and opted for water and herbal teas. Within weeks, Rose began to feel a noticeable difference. Her energy levels soared, her digestion improved, and she started to lose weight steadily.

Rose's story is a powerful example of how dietary changes can transform your life. It shows that eating right and drinking pure isn't just about following a diet; it's about adopting a lifestyle that promotes overall well-being. This book, "Eat Right, Drink Pure, Be Well: A Comprehensive Guide To Healthy Drinking and Eating," aims to guide you on a similar journey toward better health.

Goals of the Book

The main goal of this book is to provide you with the knowledge and tools you need to make healthier food and drink choices. We will explore the basics of nutrition, debunk common myths, and offer practical advice on how to eat and drink in a way that supports your body and mind. By the end of this book, you will have a clear understanding of how to create a balanced, nutritious diet that suits your lifestyle and health goals.

Understanding Nutrition

Nutrition is the foundation of good health. It involves more than just counting calories or following the latest diet trends. Good nutrition is about giving your body the right balance of nutrients to function properly. These nutrients include carbohydrates, proteins, fats, vitamins, and minerals. Each plays a vital role in maintaining your health and well-being.

Carbohydrates are your body's main source of energy. However, not all carbs are created equal. Whole grains, fruits, and vegetables provide complex carbs that give you sustained energy and are packed with fiber and nutrients. On the other hand, refined carbs like white bread and sugary snacks can cause energy spikes and crashes and are often low in essential nutrients.

Proteins are the building blocks of your body. They are crucial for repairing tissues, making enzymes and hormones, and supporting overall growth and development. Incorporating a variety of protein sources, including plant-based options like beans and nuts, can help ensure you get all the essential amino acids your body needs.

Fats are essential for brain health, hormone production, and absorbing certain vitamins. Healthy fats, such as those found in avocados, nuts, and olive oil, can help protect your heart and support overall health. Avoiding trans fats and limiting saturated fats can reduce your risk of heart disease and other chronic conditions.

Vitamins and minerals are micronutrients that play a critical role in maintaining bodily functions. They support your immune system, help your body produce energy, and ensure your organs work properly. Eating a diverse range of foods, particularly fruits and vegetables, helps you get a broad spectrum of these essential nutrients.

Debunking Myths

There are many myths about diet and nutrition that can lead to confusion and poor health choices. This book aims to clear up some of the most common misconceptions.

Myth 1: All fats are bad. Not all fats are created equal. While trans fats and excessive saturated fats can be harmful, healthy fats are essential for your body. Including sources of unsaturated fats, like fish, nuts, and seeds, can improve heart health and overall well-being.

Myth 2: Carbs make you gain weight. Carbohydrates are an important part of a balanced diet. The key is to choose complex carbs over refined ones. Whole grains, fruits, and vegetables provide fiber and nutrients that support health and help manage weight.

Myth 3: You need to eat less to lose weight. Weight management isn't just about eating less; it's about eating smart. Focusing on nutrient-dense foods that fill you up and provide essential nutrients can help you lose weight and maintain it without feeling deprived.

Myth 4: Supplements can replace a healthy diet. While supplements can help fill nutritional gaps, they cannot replace the benefits of a varied and balanced diet. Whole foods provide a combination of nutrients and other beneficial compounds that work together to support your health.

Practical Advice for Eating Right

Eating right involves more than just choosing the right foods; it's also about how you prepare and enjoy them. Here are some practical tips to help you get started:

Plan Your Meals: Planning your meals in advance can help you make healthier choices and avoid last-minute, unhealthy options. Create a weekly meal plan that includes a variety of foods from all the food groups.

Cook at Home: Cooking at home allows you to control the ingredients and preparation methods. Try new recipes and experiment with different flavors and cooking techniques to keep your meals interesting.

Eat Mindfully: Pay attention to what and how much you're eating. Slow down and savor each bite, and listen to your body's hunger and fullness cues.

Stay Hydrated: Drinking enough water is essential for overall health. Aim for at least 8 cups of water a day, and choose water or herbal teas over sugary drinks.

Snack Smart: Choose healthy snacks like fruits, vegetables, nuts, and yogurt. Avoid processed snacks that are high in sugar and unhealthy fats.

Drinking Pure

Just as important as what you eat is what you drink. Many people consume a significant number of empty calories and unhealthy substances through their beverages. Here's how to make healthier drink choices:

Choose Water: Water is the best choice for staying hydrated. It has no calories and supports all of your body's functions.

Limit Sugary Drinks: Beverages like soda, energy drinks, and sweetened coffee drinks can be high in added sugars and calories. Cutting back on these drinks can significantly improve your health.

Enjoy Herbal Teas: Herbal teas are a great way to add flavor without added sugars or calories. They also offer various health benefits depending on the herbs used.

Avoid Excessive Alcohol: While moderate alcohol consumption can be part of a healthy diet, excessive drinking can lead to numerous health problems. Stick to recommended guidelines, which suggest up to one drink per day for women and up to two drinks per day for men.

Balancing Your Diet

Creating a balanced diet doesn't have to be complicated. It's about including a variety of foods that provide the nutrients your body needs. Here are some key principles:

Variety is Key: Eating a wide range of foods ensures you get a broad spectrum of nutrients. Try to include different colors and types of fruits and vegetables in your meals.

Portion Control: Be mindful of portion sizes to avoid overeating. Using smaller plates and paying attention to serving sizes can help.

Include All Food Groups: Make sure your meals include a balance of carbohydrates, proteins, fats, and plenty of fruits and vegetables.

Moderation: It's okay to enjoy your favorite treats in moderation. The key is to focus on overall patterns of healthy eating rather than perfection.

Rose's Journey

Rose's transformation didn't happen overnight. It was a gradual process of learning, adapting, and making better choices. She discovered that eating right and drinking pure was not about strict rules or deprivation, but about nurturing her body and enjoying her food. Rose found joy in trying new recipes, exploring different foods, and seeing the positive changes in her health.

Her story is a testament to the power of a healthy diet. It shows that anyone can make positive changes, no matter where they start. This book is here to guide you on your own journey to better health. Whether you're looking to lose weight, boost your energy, or simply feel better, the information and tips in this book can help you achieve your goals.

"Eat Right, Drink Pure, Be Well: A Comprehensive Guide To Healthy Drinking and Eating" is designed to be a practical and accessible resource for anyone looking to improve their health through better nutrition. With clear explanations, debunked myths, and practical tips, this book aims to empower you to make informed choices that support your well-being.

Remember, healthy eating is a journey, not a destination. It's about making small, sustainable changes that add up over time. As you read through the chapters and implement the advice, you'll start to see and feel the benefits of a balanced, nutritious diet. Continue reading.

Chapter 1: Understanding Nutrition Basics

What is Nutrition?

Nutrition is all about how food affects our bodies and health. It involves understanding what we eat and how it helps us live and grow. Our bodies need different types of nutrients to function properly. These nutrients are divided into two main categories: macronutrients and micronutrients.

Macronutrients

Macronutrients are the nutrients our bodies need in larger amounts. They provide the energy we need to perform everyday activities and stay healthy. There are three main types of macronutrients: carbohydrates, proteins, and fats.

Carbohydrates: Carbs are the body's main source of energy. They break down into glucose, which fuels our cells, especially our brain and muscles.

Proteins: Proteins are essential for building and repairing tissues, making enzymes and hormones, and supporting overall growth and development.

Fats: Fats provide a concentrated source of energy, help absorb certain vitamins, and are necessary for building cell membranes and producing hormones.

Micronutrients

Micronutrients are needed in smaller amounts but are still crucial for good health. They include vitamins and minerals.

Vitamins: These are organic compounds that our bodies need to function properly. Each vitamin has a specific role, such as supporting the immune system, aiding in the production of energy, and maintaining healthy skin and bones.

Minerals: These are inorganic elements that help with various bodily functions, such as building strong bones, transmitting nerve impulses, and maintaining a normal heart rhythm.

The Role of Carbohydrates

Carbohydrates are one of the main sources of energy for our bodies. They are found in foods like bread, pasta, rice, fruits, vegetables, and dairy products. Not all carbohydrates are the same, and understanding the difference between good and bad carbs can help us make healthier choices.

Good Carbohydrates

Good carbs, also known as complex carbohydrates, provide long-lasting energy and are rich in fiber, vitamins, and minerals. They are found in whole, unprocessed foods. Examples include:
Whole Grains: Foods like brown rice, quinoa, oats, and whole wheat bread.
Fruits and Vegetables: Fresh produce that is high in fiber and nutrients.
Legumes: Beans, lentils, and peas are great sources of complex carbs and protein.

Complex carbs break down slowly, keeping our blood sugar levels stable and providing a steady source of energy. They also help with digestion and can prevent constipation.

Bad Carbohydrates

Bad carbs, also known as simple carbohydrates or refined carbs, provide quick energy but are often stripped of their nutrients and fiber. They can cause rapid spikes and drops in blood sugar levels, leading to energy crashes and increased hunger. Examples include:
Sugary Snacks: Candy, cookies, and cakes.
Sugary Drinks: Sodas, energy drinks, and sweetened fruit juices.

Refined Grains: White bread, white rice, and pasta made from refined flour.

Eating too many bad carbs can lead to weight gain, type 2 diabetes, and other health issues. It's best to limit these foods and focus on consuming more complex carbs.

Fats and Your Health

Fats often get a bad reputation, but they are an essential part of a healthy diet. Fats provide energy, support cell growth, protect our organs, and help our bodies absorb vitamins. There are different types of fats, and some are healthier than others.

Beneficial Fats

Beneficial fats, also known as healthy fats, can improve heart health and support overall well-being. They are found in natural, unprocessed foods. Examples include:

Monounsaturated Fats: Found in olive oil, avocados, and nuts.

Polyunsaturated Fats: Found in fatty fish (like salmon), flaxseeds, and walnuts. These include omega-3 and omega-6 fatty acids, which are essential for brain function and cell growth.

These fats can help reduce bad cholesterol levels, lower the risk of heart disease, and provide anti-inflammatory benefits.

Harmful Fats

Harmful fats, also known as unhealthy fats, can increase the risk of heart disease, stroke, and other health problems. They are often found in processed and fried foods. Examples include:
Saturated Fats: Found in red meat, butter, cheese, and other animal products. While small amounts are okay, too much can raise cholesterol levels.
Trans Fats: Found in margarine, shortening, and many processed foods like cookies, cakes, and fast food. These fats are the worst for health and should be avoided as much as possible.

Eating a diet high in unhealthy fats can lead to weight gain, clogged arteries, and increased risk of chronic diseases. It's important to choose healthy fats and limit or avoid unhealthy ones.

Proteins for Power

Proteins are vital for our bodies. They help build and repair tissues, make enzymes and hormones, and support immune function. Proteins are made up of smaller units called amino acids. Our bodies can produce some amino acids, but others, known as essential amino acids, must come from our diet.

Choosing the Right Proteins

Proteins come from both animal and plant sources. It's important to include a variety of protein sources in your diet to get all the essential amino acids.

Animal Proteins: These are complete proteins, meaning they contain all the essential amino acids. Examples include meat, poultry, fish, eggs, and dairy products. While these are good sources of protein, it's best to choose lean cuts of meat and low-fat dairy to reduce intake of saturated fats.

Plant Proteins: These are often incomplete proteins, meaning they may lack one or more essential amino acids. However, by eating a variety of plant proteins, you can get all the amino acids you need. Examples include beans, lentils, tofu, nuts, seeds, and whole grains.

Incorporating plant-based proteins into your diet can provide additional benefits like fiber, vitamins, and minerals, while also reducing the intake of unhealthy fats.

Vitamins and Minerals

Vitamins and minerals are essential nutrients that our bodies need to function properly. They play a role in many bodily processes, including growth, development, and maintaining health.

Vitamins

Vitamins are organic compounds that help with various functions in the body. There are 13 essential vitamins, each with specific roles:

Vitamin A: Important for vision, immune function, and skin health. Found in carrots, sweet potatoes, and spinach.

Vitamin C: Helps with the growth and repair of tissues, boosts the immune system, and acts as an antioxidant. Found in citrus fruits, strawberries, and bell peppers.

Vitamin D: Helps with calcium absorption, bone health, and immune function. Found in sunlight, fatty fish, and fortified dairy products.

Vitamin E: Acts as an antioxidant, supports immune function, and helps with skin health. Found in nuts, seeds, and green leafy vegetables.

Vitamin K: Essential for blood clotting and bone health. Found in green leafy vegetables, broccoli, and Brussels sprouts.

B Vitamins: Includes a group of vitamins (B1, B2, B3, B5, B6, B7, B9, and B12) that help with energy production, brain function, and cell metabolism. Found in whole grains, meat, eggs, and dairy.

Minerals

Minerals are inorganic elements that our bodies need to function properly. Some important minerals include:

Calcium: Necessary for strong bones and teeth, muscle function, and nerve signaling. Found in dairy products, leafy greens, and fortified plant-based milks.

Iron: Helps with the production of hemoglobin, which carries oxygen in the blood. Found in red meat, beans, and fortified cereals.

Magnesium: Supports muscle and nerve function, blood sugar control, and bone health. Found in nuts, seeds, and whole grains.

Potassium: Helps with muscle function, nerve signaling, and balancing fluids in the body. Found in bananas, potatoes, and beans.

Zinc: Important for immune function, wound healing, and DNA synthesis. Found in meat, shellfish, and legumes.

Understanding the basics of nutrition is the first step towards making healthier choices. By focusing on the quality of the foods you eat and ensuring a balance of macronutrients and micronutrients, you can support your overall health and well-being.

Here are some tips to help you put this knowledge into practice:

Eat a Variety of Foods: Include different types of fruits, vegetables, whole grains, proteins, and healthy fats in your diet to ensure you get a wide range of nutrients.

Choose Whole Foods: Opt for minimally processed foods that are close to their natural state. Whole foods provide more nutrients and fiber compared to processed foods.

Balance Your Plate: Aim to fill half your plate with fruits and vegetables, a quarter with lean proteins, and a quarter with whole grains. Add a small amount of healthy fats for a balanced meal.

Stay Hydrated: Drink plenty of water throughout the day to support your body's functions. Limit sugary drinks and alcohol.

Practice Portion Control: Be mindful of portion sizes to avoid overeating. Using smaller plates and bowls can help with portion control.

Plan Ahead: Plan your meals and snacks in advance to make healthier choices and avoid the temptation of unhealthy options.

Listen to Your Body: Pay attention to your hunger and fullness cues. Eat when you're hungry and stop when you're satisfied.

By making small, sustainable changes to your eating habits, you can improve your health and feel better every day. Remember, nutrition is not about perfection, but about making better choices more often.

Nutrition is the foundation of good health. By understanding the basics of macronutrients and micronutrients, and making informed choices about the foods you eat, you can support your body's needs and improve your overall well-being. Carbohydrates, fats, proteins, vitamins, and minerals all play vital roles in maintaining health, and choosing the right types of these nutrients can make a significant difference.

In the following chapters, we will dive deeper into specific aspects of a healthy diet, explore practical tips for meal planning and preparation, and provide delicious recipes to help you enjoy nutritious foods every day. By the end of this book, you will have the tools and knowledge you need to eat right, drink pure, and be well.

Chapter 2: Examining the USDA Dietary Guidelines

Understanding how dietary guidelines have evolved over time and identifying common misconceptions is essential for making healthier food choices. In this chapter, we'll explore the history of the USDA dietary guidelines, examine where they may have gone wrong, and look at what modern research suggests for optimal nutrition.

Historical Perspective: The Evolution of Dietary Guidelines

Dietary guidelines are recommendations aimed at helping people make healthier food choices. The United States Department of Agriculture (USDA) has been providing these guidelines for over a century. Let's take a look at how they have changed over the years.

Early Guidelines (1916-1940s)

The USDA's first dietary guidelines were introduced in 1916, focusing on food groups and the importance of a balanced diet. These early guidelines emphasized eating a variety of foods to ensure adequate nutrient intake. The five food groups were:

- Milk and meat
- Cereals and grains
- Vegetables and fruits
- Fats and fatty foods
- Sugars and sugary foods

During the 1940s, the focus shifted to preventing nutritional deficiencies, especially during World War II when food rationing was common. The guidelines emphasized the importance of eating nutrient-dense foods to ensure Americans received essential vitamins and minerals.

The Food Pyramid (1992)

In 1992, the USDA introduced the Food Guide Pyramid, a visual representation of how different food groups should be balanced. The pyramid had six sections:

- Grains (bread, cereal, rice, pasta)
- Vegetables
- Fruits
- Dairy (milk, yogurt, cheese)
- Protein (meat, poultry, fish, beans, eggs, nuts)
- Fats, oils, and sweets

The pyramid suggested a high intake of grains (6-11 servings per day) and limited consumption of fats and sweets. This approach aimed to promote a low-fat diet, which was believed to reduce the risk of heart disease and obesity.

MyPlate (2011)

In 2011, the USDA replaced the Food Guide Pyramid with MyPlate, a simpler visual guide that divided a plate into four sections:
- Vegetables
- Fruits
- Grains
- Protein

A smaller circle next to the plate represented dairy. MyPlate aimed to provide a more straightforward guide to healthy eating, emphasizing portion control and the importance of including a variety of food groups in every meal.

Common Misconceptions: What the USDA Got Wrong

While the USDA dietary guidelines have evolved with the intention of improving public health, they have faced criticism for various reasons. Here are some common misconceptions and issues with these guidelines.

Overemphasis on Grains

One of the main criticisms of the USDA guidelines is the overemphasis on grains, particularly refined grains. The Food Guide Pyramid recommended 6-11 servings of grains per day, which led many people to consume large amounts of bread, pasta, and other refined grain products.

Refined grains are stripped of fiber and essential nutrients during processing, which can lead to spikes in blood sugar levels and increased hunger. This can contribute to weight gain and a higher risk of developing type 2 diabetes and other chronic diseases.

Low-Fat Diet Emphasis

The guidelines have long promoted a low-fat diet, suggesting that reducing fat intake would lower the risk of heart disease. However, this advice often led people to replace fats with refined carbohydrates and sugars, which can have negative health effects.

Research has shown that not all fats are bad. Healthy fats, such as those found in avocados, nuts, seeds, and fatty fish, are essential for brain health, hormone production, and overall well-being. Overemphasizing low-fat diets may have inadvertently contributed to an increase in obesity and metabolic disorders.

Lack of Focus on Whole Foods

The USDA guidelines have sometimes been criticized for not emphasizing whole, unprocessed foods enough. Instead, they often focused on nutrient content, which led to the promotion of processed foods that were fortified with vitamins and minerals but still lacked the overall health benefits of whole foods.
Whole foods, such as fruits, vegetables, whole grains, and lean proteins, provide a wide range of nutrients, fiber, and beneficial compounds that work together to support health. Processed foods, even when fortified, cannot replicate the benefits of whole foods.

Inadequate Attention to Individual Needs

The guidelines have typically provided broad recommendations that may not address individual dietary needs. Factors such as age, gender, activity level, and existing health conditions can significantly impact nutritional requirements. One-size-fits-all guidelines may not be suitable for everyone, leading to suboptimal dietary choices for some individuals.

Evidence-Based Nutrition: What Modern Research Shows

Modern research has provided new insights into nutrition and health, challenging some of the traditional recommendations. Here's what current evidence suggests about a healthy diet.

Balanced Macronutrients

Instead of focusing on low-fat or low-carb diets, current research emphasizes the importance of a balanced intake of macronutrients—carbohydrates, proteins, and fats. Each of these nutrients plays a crucial role in maintaining health, and the key is to choose high-quality sources.

Carbohydrates: Opt for complex carbohydrates, such as whole grains, fruits, and vegetables, which provide fiber and essential nutrients.

Proteins: Include a variety of protein sources, both animal and plant-based, to ensure you get all the essential amino acids.

Fats: Incorporate healthy fats from sources like avocados, nuts, seeds, and fatty fish, while limiting saturated and trans fats.

Importance of Fiber

Fiber is essential for digestive health, blood sugar control, and weight management. Foods high in fiber, such as whole grains, legumes, fruits, and vegetables, should be a significant part of your diet. Fiber helps you feel full, supports healthy digestion, and can reduce the risk of chronic diseases like heart disease and type 2 diabetes.

Role of Healthy Fats

Healthy fats are vital for overall health. Monounsaturated fats (found in olive oil, avocados, and nuts) and polyunsaturated fats (found in fish, flaxseeds, and walnuts) have been shown to reduce inflammation and improve heart health. Omega-3 fatty acids, in particular, are crucial for brain function and reducing the risk of heart disease.

Protein Quality

Protein is essential for building and repairing tissues, making enzymes and hormones, and supporting immune function. It's important to choose high-quality protein sources, such as lean meats, fish, eggs, dairy, beans, lentils, tofu, and quinoa. Including a mix of animal and plant-based proteins can provide a broad spectrum of nutrients.

Whole Foods vs. Processed Foods

Whole foods should form the basis of a healthy diet. These include fresh fruits and vegetables, whole grains, lean proteins, and healthy fats. Whole foods provide a wide range of nutrients, fiber, and beneficial compounds that processed foods lack. Processed foods, on the other hand, often contain added sugars, unhealthy fats, and artificial ingredients. They can contribute to weight gain, inflammation, and chronic diseases. Limiting processed foods and focusing on whole foods can significantly improve your health.

Individualized Nutrition

Modern research recognizes that individual nutritional needs can vary widely. Factors such as age, gender, activity level, and health status all influence dietary requirements. Personalized nutrition plans that take these factors into account can be more effective than one-size-fits-all guidelines.

Mindful Eating

Mindful eating involves paying attention to what you eat, savoring each bite, and listening to your body's hunger and fullness cues. This practice can help you make healthier food choices, enjoy your meals more, and avoid overeating. Mindful eating encourages a healthier relationship with food.

Practical Tips for Applying Modern Nutrition Research

Based on the insights from modern nutrition research, here are some practical tips to help you make healthier food choices and improve your overall well-being.

Embrace a Balanced Diet

Include a variety of foods: Aim to include different types of fruits, vegetables, whole grains, proteins, and healthy fats in your diet.

Balance your macronutrients: Ensure you're getting a good mix of carbohydrates, proteins, and fats from high-quality sources.

Focus on nutrient density: Choose foods that provide a lot of nutrients for relatively few calories. These include vegetables, fruits, lean proteins, and whole grains.

Choose Whole Foods

Opt for fresh produce: Fresh fruits and vegetables are rich in vitamins, minerals, and fiber. They should be a staple in your diet.
Select whole grains: Choose whole grains like brown rice, quinoa, and whole wheat over refined grains.
Pick lean proteins: Lean meats, fish, eggs, beans, and lentils are excellent protein sources that provide essential nutrients without too much unhealthy fat.
Incorporate healthy fats: Avocados, nuts, seeds, and olive oil are great sources of healthy fats that support heart health and overall well-being.

Limit Processed Foods

Read labels: Check the ingredient lists and nutrition labels on packaged foods. Avoid products with added sugars, trans fats, and artificial ingredients.
Cook at home: Preparing meals at home gives you control over the ingredients and cooking methods, allowing you to make healthier choices.
Snack smart: Choose healthy snacks like fruits, vegetables, nuts, and yogurt instead of processed snacks that are high in sugar and unhealthy fats.

Personalize Your Diet

Listen to your body: Pay attention to how different foods make you feel. Adjust your diet based on your energy levels, digestion, and overall well-being.

Consider your lifestyle: Tailor your diet to your activity level, age, and any specific health conditions you may have. For example, athletes may need more protein, while older adults might require more calcium and vitamin D.

Seek professional advice: Consult with a registered dietitian or nutritionist to develop a personalized nutrition plan that meets your unique needs.

Practice Mindful Eating

Eat slowly: Take your time to chew your food thoroughly and savor each bite. This can help you enjoy your meals more and prevent overeating.

Pay attention to hunger and fullness: Listen to your body's signals and eat when you're hungry. Stop eating when you feel satisfied, not overly full.

Avoid distractions: Try to eat without distractions like TV or smartphones. Focus on your meal and the experience of eating.

The USDA dietary guidelines have evolved over time, aiming to help people make healthier food choices. However, they have faced criticism for overemphasizing certain food groups, promoting low-fat diets, and not focusing enough on whole foods. Modern nutrition research provides new insights that challenge some traditional recommendations and emphasize the importance of a balanced diet, whole foods, and personalized nutrition.

By understanding the historical perspective of dietary guidelines, recognizing common misconceptions, and applying evidence-based nutrition principles, you can make more informed food choices that support your health and well-being. Remember, healthy eating is not about strict rules or deprivation; it's about making better choices more often and finding a balance that works for you.

Chapter 3: Weight Control and Longevity

The Weight Connection: How Weight Impacts Health

Maintaining a healthy weight is crucial for overall well-being and longevity. Your weight can significantly impact your physical health, mental health, and quality of life. Let's explore how weight influences different aspects of health.

Physical Health

Heart Disease and Stroke: Excess weight, especially around the abdomen, increases the risk of heart disease and stroke. Fat deposits around the midsection are associated with higher levels of bad cholesterol and triglycerides, which can clog arteries. This leads to higher blood pressure and greater strain on the heart.

Type 2 Diabetes: Being overweight or obese is a major risk factor for developing type 2 diabetes. Excess body fat, particularly around the belly, makes it harder for your body to use insulin properly. This leads to insulin resistance, where your cells do not respond well to insulin, causing blood sugar levels to rise. Over time, this can damage organs and lead to serious complications like kidney failure, blindness, and nerve damage.

High Blood Pressure: Carrying extra weight puts additional strain on your arteries. As your body works harder to circulate blood, your blood pressure increases. High blood pressure can damage your arteries over time, increasing the risk of heart attack, stroke, and kidney disease.

Joint Problems: Extra weight puts more pressure on your joints, particularly in the knees, hips, and lower back. This can lead to joint pain and conditions like osteoarthritis, where the cartilage that cushions the joints wears down, causing pain and stiffness.

Respiratory Issues: Obesity can lead to breathing problems like sleep apnea, a condition where breathing repeatedly stops and starts during sleep. Extra fat around the neck can block airways, leading to interrupted sleep and decreased oxygen supply to the body.

Certain Cancers: Being overweight or obese increases the risk of several types of cancer, including breast, colon, endometrial, and kidney cancer. Excess body fat can lead to chronic inflammation, hormonal imbalances, and insulin resistance, all of which can promote cancer growth.

Reproductive Health: Excess weight can affect reproductive health in both men and women. In women, it can lead to irregular menstrual cycles, polycystic ovary syndrome (PCOS), and complications during pregnancy. In men, obesity can reduce sperm quality and fertility.

Immune System Function: Obesity can weaken the immune system, making it harder for the body to fight off infections. This is due to chronic inflammation caused by excess fat, which impairs immune function.

Mental Health

Depression and Anxiety: There is a strong link between obesity and mental health issues like depression and anxiety. The stigma and discrimination faced by people who are overweight can lead to low self-esteem and social isolation. Additionally, the physical discomfort and health problems associated with obesity can contribute to mental health struggles.

Stress: Carrying excess weight can lead to higher levels of stress. The pressure to lose weight, combined with the physical discomfort of being overweight, can create a cycle of stress and emotional eating, which makes weight management even more challenging.

Body Image: Being overweight can negatively affect body image and self-esteem. Constantly comparing oneself to societal standards of beauty can lead to feelings of inadequacy and shame, which can further impact mental health and overall well-being.

Healthy Weight Management: Strategies to Control Weight Effectively

Achieving and maintaining a healthy weight is about finding a balance that works for your body and lifestyle. Here are some strategies to help you manage your weight effectively.

Balanced Diet: A balanced diet is crucial for weight management. It provides your body with the nutrients it needs to function properly while helping you maintain a healthy weight.

Eat a Variety of Foods: Include a wide range of foods in your diet to ensure you get all the essential nutrients. Focus on fruits, vegetables, whole grains, lean proteins, and healthy fats. Each food group provides different nutrients that your body needs.

Focus on Whole Foods: Choose whole, unprocessed foods as much as possible. Whole foods are naturally rich in nutrients and fiber, which help you feel full and satisfied. They also contain fewer added sugars, unhealthy fats, and artificial ingredients compared to processed foods.

Control Portions: Be mindful of portion sizes. Eating large portions can lead to consuming more calories than your body needs, which can result in weight gain. Use smaller plates, measure portions, and listen to your body's hunger and fullness cues to avoid overeating.

Limit Added Sugars and Refined Carbohydrates

Foods high in added sugars and refined carbohydrates can cause rapid spikes in blood sugar levels, leading to increased hunger and cravings. These foods are also often high in calories but low in nutrients. Limit sugary snacks, sodas, and refined grains like white bread and pasta.

Stay Hydrated: Drinking enough water is important for weight management. Sometimes, our bodies can mistake thirst for hunger, leading to unnecessary snacking. Aim to drink at least 8 cups of water a day and choose water over sugary drinks.

Regular Physical Activity: Exercise is a key component of weight management. It helps burn calories, build muscle, and improve overall health. Here are some tips for incorporating physical activity into your routine.

Find Activities You Enjoy: The best exercise is one you enjoy and can stick with long-term. Whether it's walking, running, swimming, dancing, or playing a sport, find activities that you look forward to doing.

Aim for Consistency: Consistency is more important than intensity. Aim for at least 150 minutes of moderate-intensity aerobic activity, such as brisk walking, per week. You can break this down into shorter sessions throughout the week.

Include Strength Training: Strength training exercises, such as lifting weights or doing bodyweight exercises, help build muscle and increase metabolism. Aim to include strength training at least twice a week.

Make Exercise a Habit: Incorporate physical activity into your daily routine. Take the stairs instead of the elevator, walk or bike to work, or do a quick workout during lunch breaks. Making small changes can add up over time.

Mindful Eating: Mindful eating involves paying attention to what and how you eat. It helps you develop a healthier relationship with food and can aid in weight management.

Eat Slowly: Take your time to chew your food thoroughly and savor each bite. Eating slowly gives your body time to signal when it's full, helping you avoid overeating.

Listen to Your Body: Pay attention to your body's hunger and fullness cues. Eat when you're hungry and stop when you're satisfied. Avoid eating out of boredom, stress, or habit.

Avoid Distractions: Try to eat without distractions like TV or smartphones. Focus on your meal and the experience of eating. This can help you enjoy your food more and prevent overeating.

Plan Your Meals: Planning your meals in advance can help you make healthier choices and avoid last-minute, unhealthy options. Create a weekly meal plan that includes a variety of foods from all the food groups.

Healthy Snacking: Choose healthy snacks that provide nutrients and help keep you full between meals. Fruits, vegetables, nuts, and yogurt are good options. Avoid processed snacks that are high in sugar and unhealthy fats.

Lifestyle Changes: Incorporating Exercise and Mindful Eating

In addition to healthy eating and regular physical activity, making other lifestyle changes can support weight management and overall health.

Prioritize Sleep: Getting enough sleep is crucial for weight management and overall health. Poor sleep can disrupt hormones that control hunger and appetite, making it harder to maintain a healthy weight.

Establish a Sleep Routine: Try to go to bed and wake up at the same time every day, even on weekends. This helps regulate your body's internal clock and improve sleep quality.

Create a Relaxing Sleep Environment: Make your bedroom a calm and comfortable space. Keep it cool, dark, and quiet. Avoid screens and bright lights before bedtime, as they can interfere with your sleep.

Limit Caffeine and Alcohol: Caffeine and alcohol can disrupt sleep patterns. Try to limit their consumption, especially in the hours leading up to bedtime.

Manage Stress: Chronic stress can lead to weight gain and other health issues. Finding healthy ways to manage stress is important for overall well-being.

Practice Relaxation Techniques

Activities like yoga, meditation, and deep breathing exercises can help reduce stress levels and promote relaxation.

Stay Active: Regular physical activity is a great way to manage stress. Exercise releases endorphins, which are natural mood boosters.

Connect with Others: Spending time with friends and family can provide emotional support and help reduce stress. Social connections are important for mental health.

Pursue Hobbies: Engaging in activities you enjoy can help take your mind off stress and improve your mood. Whether it's reading, gardening, or painting, find hobbies that bring you joy.

Maintaining a healthy weight is essential for overall health and longevity. Excess weight can lead to a range of health problems, including heart disease, diabetes, and joint issues, while also impacting mental health and quality of life. Achieving and maintaining a healthy weight involves a combination of healthy eating, regular physical activity, and mindful lifestyle choices.

By focusing on a balanced diet, staying active, practicing mindful eating, and making other positive lifestyle changes, you can improve your health, feel better, and increase your chances of living a longer, healthier life. Remember, weight management is not about perfection but about making sustainable, healthy choices that support your overall well-being.

Chapter 4: The Best Carbohydrates for Your Diet

Carbohydrates are a crucial part of a healthy diet. They are the body's primary source of energy, especially for the brain and muscles. However, not all carbohydrates are created equal. In this chapter, we will explore the differences between whole grains and refined grains, the importance of fiber-rich foods, and the glycemic index's role in blood sugar management.

Whole Grains vs. Refined Grains: Making the Right Choice

Carbohydrates come in many forms, but they are generally classified into two main types: whole grains and refined grains. Understanding the differences between these two can help you make healthier choices for your diet.

Whole Grains: Whole grains are grains that contain all parts of the grain kernel – the bran, germ, and endosperm. Because they include all these parts, they retain more nutrients and fiber. Common whole grains include:

- Brown Rice
- Quinoa
- Oats
- Whole Wheat
- Barley
- Millet
- Buckwheat

Whole grains are rich in essential nutrients such as B vitamins, iron, magnesium, and selenium. They also provide dietary fiber, which is important for digestive health.

Benefits of Whole Grains

Nutrient-Rich: Whole grains are packed with essential nutrients that help maintain overall health.

High in Fiber: The fiber in whole grains helps regulate digestion, maintain healthy blood sugar levels, and keep you feeling full longer.

Heart Health: Consuming whole grains can reduce the risk of heart disease by lowering cholesterol levels and improving blood pressure.

Weight Management: The fiber in whole grains can help with weight management by promoting a feeling of fullness and reducing overeating.

Incorporating Whole Grains into Your Diet

Breakfast: Start your day with a bowl of oatmeal or a slice of whole wheat toast.

Lunch: Add quinoa or brown rice to your salads or use whole grain bread for sandwiches.

Dinner: Replace refined grains with whole grains in your meals. For example, use whole wheat pasta or serve your stir-fry with barley.

Snacks: Choose whole grain snacks like popcorn or whole grain crackers.

Refined Grains

Refined grains have been processed to remove the bran and germ, leaving only the endosperm. This process strips away many of the grain's nutrients and fiber. Common refined grains include:

- White Rice
- White Bread
- Pasta made from refined flour
- Most breakfast cereals
- Pastries and baked goods made with white flour

Refined grains are often enriched, meaning some nutrients are added back after processing. However, they still lack the fiber and many of the original nutrients found in whole grains.

Drawbacks of Refined Grains

Low in Nutrients: The refining process removes many essential nutrients.
Low in Fiber: Without the bran and germ, refined grains have significantly less fiber, which can lead to digestive issues and increased hunger.
Blood Sugar Spikes: Refined grains can cause rapid spikes in blood sugar levels, followed by crashes, leading to increased hunger and cravings.
Weight Gain: The lack of fiber and rapid digestion of refined grains can contribute to overeating and weight gain.

Reducing Refined Grains in Your Diet

Read Labels: Look for products labeled as "100% whole grain" or "whole wheat." Avoid products with refined flour as the first ingredient.
Cook at Home: Prepare meals using whole grains instead of relying on processed foods.
Swap Ingredients: Replace white rice with brown rice, white bread with whole wheat bread, and regular pasta with whole wheat pasta.

Fiber-Rich Foods: Benefits and Sources

Fiber is a type of carbohydrate that the body cannot digest. It is found in plant-based foods and is essential for maintaining good health. There are two main types of fiber: soluble and insoluble.

Soluble Fiber

Soluble fiber dissolves in water to form a gel-like substance. It can help lower blood cholesterol and glucose levels. Foods rich in soluble fiber include:

- Oats
- Beans and legumes
- Fruits (such as apples, oranges, and berries)
- Vegetables (such as carrots and Brussels sprouts)
- Barley
- Psyllium

Insoluble Fiber

Insoluble fiber does not dissolve in water and helps add bulk to the stool, promoting regular bowel movements. Foods rich in insoluble fiber include:

- Whole grains
- Nuts and seeds

- Vegetables (such as broccoli, cauliflower, and green beans)
- Wheat bran

Benefits of Fiber

Digestive Health: Fiber helps regulate bowel movements, preventing constipation and promoting a healthy digestive system.

Heart Health: Soluble fiber can help lower cholesterol levels, reducing the risk of heart disease.

Blood Sugar Control: Fiber slows the absorption of sugar, helping to control blood sugar levels and reduce the risk of type 2 diabetes.

Weight Management: Fiber adds bulk to your diet, helping you feel full longer and reducing the likelihood of overeating.

Increasing Fiber in Your Diet

Eat More Fruits and Vegetables: Aim for at least five servings of fruits and vegetables each day. Choose whole fruits over fruit juices for more fiber.

Choose Whole Grains: Replace refined grains with whole grains, such as brown rice, whole wheat bread, and oatmeal.

Add Legumes: Include beans, lentils, and other legumes in your meals. They are excellent sources of fiber and protein.

Snack on Nuts and Seeds: Nuts and seeds are not only rich in fiber but also provide healthy fats and protein.

Incorporate Fiber-Rich Foods into Recipes: Add vegetables to soups and stews, include beans in salads, and mix flaxseeds or chia seeds into yogurt or smoothies.

Glycemic Index: Understanding Its Impact on Blood Sugar

The glycemic index (GI) is a measure of how quickly a carbohydrate-containing food raises blood sugar levels. Foods are ranked on a scale from 0 to 100, with pure glucose scoring 100. Understanding the glycemic index can help you make better choices for maintaining stable blood sugar levels.

Low GI Foods

Low GI foods have a GI score of 55 or less. These foods cause a slower, more gradual rise in blood sugar levels. Examples of low GI foods include:

- Non-starchy vegetables (such as broccoli, spinach, and peppers)
- Most fruits (such as apples, oranges, and berries)

- Whole grains (such as barley, quinoa, and oats)
- Legumes (such as beans, lentils, and chickpeas)
- Nuts and seeds

Benefits of Low GI Foods

Stable Blood Sugar Levels: Low GI foods help prevent blood sugar spikes and crashes, providing a more stable source of energy.

Reduced Risk of Diabetes: Eating low GI foods can help lower the risk of developing type 2 diabetes by improving insulin sensitivity.

Improved Weight Management: Low GI foods can help control appetite and reduce cravings, making it easier to manage weight.

Heart Health: Consuming low GI foods is associated with lower cholesterol levels and a reduced risk of heart disease.

High GI Foods

High GI foods have a GI score of 70 or higher. These foods cause a rapid increase in blood sugar levels. Examples of high GI foods include:

- White bread and bagels
- White rice
- Sugary cereals

- Pastries and baked goods
- Potatoes (especially when mashed or fried)
- Candy and sugary snacks

Drawbacks of High GI Foods

Blood Sugar Spikes: High GI foods can cause rapid spikes in blood sugar levels, followed by crashes. This can lead to increased hunger and cravings.

Increased Risk of Diabetes: Regularly consuming high GI foods can lead to insulin resistance and increase the risk of developing type 2 diabetes.

Weight Gain: High GI foods are often low in fiber and nutrients but high in calories, contributing to weight gain and obesity.

Heart Disease: Diets high in high GI foods are associated with higher cholesterol levels and an increased risk of heart disease.

Balancing GI in Your Diet

Combine Foods: Eating high GI foods with low GI foods can help balance blood sugar levels. For example, pair white rice with beans or add vegetables to a pasta dish.

Choose Whole Foods: Whole, unprocessed foods generally have a lower GI compared to processed foods.

Watch Portions: Be mindful of portion sizes, especially for high GI foods. Eating smaller portions can help reduce their impact on blood sugar levels.

Stay Active: Regular physical activity can help improve insulin sensitivity and manage blood sugar levels.

Making Better Carbohydrate Choices

Making informed choices about carbohydrates can have a significant impact on your health. Here are some practical tips for incorporating the best carbohydrates into your diet.

Prioritize Whole Grains

Switch to Whole Grains: Replace refined grains with whole grains like brown rice, quinoa, oats, and whole wheat bread.

Experiment with New Grains: Try different whole grains to add variety to your meals. Barley, bulgur, farro, and millet are all excellent choices.

Read Labels: Look for products labeled as "100% whole grain" or "whole wheat." Check the ingredient list to ensure whole grains are listed as the first ingredient.

Embrace Fiber-Rich Foods

Fill Half Your Plate with Fruits and Vegetables: Aim to include a variety of colors and types in your diet.

Add Legumes to Your Meals: Incorporate beans, lentils, and chickpeas into soups, stews, salads, and side dishes.

Choose Fiber-Rich Snacks: Opt for snacks like fruits, nuts, seeds, and whole grain crackers.

Manage the Glycemic Index

Combine Carbohydrates Wisely: Pair high GI foods with low GI foods to balance their impact on blood sugar levels.

Choose Low GI Options: Opt for low GI foods like non-starchy vegetables, most fruits, whole grains, and legumes.

Be Mindful of Cooking Methods: Cooking methods can affect a food's GI. For example, overcooking pasta increases its GI, while lightly cooking vegetables helps retain their low GI.

Plan and Prepare Meals

Meal Prep: Plan and prepare your meals ahead of time to ensure you have healthy, balanced options available.

Cook at Home: Cooking at home gives you control over the ingredients and portion sizes, making it easier to stick to healthy choices.

Experiment with Recipes: Try new recipes that incorporate whole grains, fiber-rich foods, and low GI ingredients. There are countless delicious and nutritious recipes available to inspire you.

Carbohydrates are an essential part of a healthy diet, but not all carbs are equal. Choosing whole grains over refined grains, incorporating fiber-rich foods, and understanding the glycemic index can help you make better carbohydrate choices. These choices can improve your overall health, help manage weight, and reduce the risk of chronic diseases.

By prioritizing whole grains, embracing fiber-rich foods, and managing the glycemic index in your diet, you can enjoy the benefits of carbohydrates while maintaining stable blood sugar levels and supporting long-term health. Remember, making small, sustainable changes to your diet can have a significant impact on your well-being.

Chapter 5: Healthy Fats You Need

Fats are an essential part of our diet. They provide energy, help absorb certain vitamins, and are crucial for brain health. However, not all fats are created equal. In this chapter, we will discuss the different types of fats, the benefits of healthy fats, and how to cook with them to make your meals healthier and more delicious.

Types of Fats: Saturated, Unsaturated, and Trans Fats

Fats can be divided into three main categories: saturated fats, unsaturated fats, and trans fats. Understanding the differences between these types of fats can help you make better dietary choices.

Saturated Fats

Saturated fats are typically solid at room temperature. They are found in animal products such as meat, butter, cheese, and full-fat dairy products. They are also present in some plant oils like coconut oil and palm oil.

Health Impact: Consuming too much saturated fat can raise the level of LDL (bad) cholesterol in your blood, which can increase the risk of heart disease and stroke. It is recommended to limit saturated fat intake to less than 10% of your total daily calories.

Unsaturated Fats

Unsaturated fats are usually liquid at room temperature and are considered healthier fats. They are found in various plant oils and fatty fish. Unsaturated fats are divided into two categories: monounsaturated fats and polyunsaturated fats.

Monounsaturated Fats: These fats are found in olive oil, avocados, nuts, and seeds. They help reduce bad cholesterol levels in your blood and lower the risk of heart disease and stroke.

Polyunsaturated Fats: These fats are found in fish, flaxseeds, walnuts, and sunflower oil. They include omega-3 and omega-6 fatty acids, which are essential for brain function and cell growth.

Health Impact: Unsaturated fats, when used in place of saturated fats and trans fats, can help reduce the risk of heart disease and improve overall health.

Trans Fats

Trans fats are artificially created through a process called hydrogenation, which solidifies liquid oils.

They are commonly found in processed foods like margarine, snack foods, and baked goods.

Health Impact: Trans fats are the most harmful type of fat. They raise bad cholesterol levels while lowering good cholesterol levels, significantly increasing the risk of heart disease and stroke. It is best to avoid trans fats entirely.

Beneficial Fats: Foods Rich in Omega-3 and Omega-6 Fatty Acids

Omega-3 and omega-6 fatty acids are types of polyunsaturated fats that are essential for good health. Our bodies cannot produce these fats, so we must get them from our diet.

Omega-3 Fatty Acids

Omega-3 fatty acids are crucial for brain health, reducing inflammation, and lowering the risk of chronic diseases such as heart disease, arthritis, and certain cancers. There are three main types of omega-3 fatty acids: ALA (alpha-linolenic acid), DHA (docosahexaenoic acid), and EPA (eicosapentaenoic acid).

Sources of Omega-3 Fatty Acids:

Fatty Fish: Salmon, mackerel, sardines, and trout are excellent sources of DHA and EPA.
Flaxseeds and Chia Seeds: These seeds are rich in ALA.
Walnuts: A good plant-based source of ALA.
Algae: Some algae supplements provide DHA, suitable for vegetarians and vegans.

Health Benefits:

Heart Health: Omega-3s help lower triglycerides, reduce blood pressure, and prevent blood clots.
Brain Health: DHA is vital for brain function and development. It may also help reduce the risk of Alzheimer's disease.
Anti-Inflammatory: Omega-3s help reduce inflammation, which can benefit conditions like arthritis.

Omega-6 Fatty Acids

Omega-6 fatty acids are also essential and play a role in brain function, skin health, and regulating metabolism. However, it is important to maintain a balance between omega-3 and omega-6 intake, as too much omega-6 can promote inflammation.

Sources of Omega-6 Fatty Acids:

Vegetable Oils: Sunflower oil, safflower oil, and soybean oil are common sources.
Nuts and Seeds: Walnuts, sunflower seeds, and pumpkin seeds contain omega-6s.
Meat and Poultry: Animal products contain omega-6 fatty acids.

Health Benefits:

Cell Function: Omega-6s are important for the structure and function of cell membranes.
Skin Health: They help keep the skin healthy and support wound healing.
Hormone Production: Omega-6 fatty acids are involved in the production of hormones that regulate various body functions.

Cooking with Healthy Fats: Tips for Everyday Meals

Incorporating healthy fats into your cooking can enhance the flavor of your meals while providing numerous health benefits. Here are some tips for using healthy fats in everyday cooking.

Choosing the Right Oils

Different oils have different properties, so it's important to choose the right oil for the type of cooking you are doing.

Olive Oil: Best for sautéing, roasting, and salad dressings. It is rich in monounsaturated fats and has a relatively low smoke point.

Avocado Oil: Good for high-heat cooking like frying and grilling due to its high smoke point. It is also rich in monounsaturated fats.

Coconut Oil: Suitable for baking and medium-heat cooking. It contains saturated fats, but it's a good option for those looking for a plant-based fat.

Canola Oil: Versatile and can be used for baking, frying, and sautéing. It has a higher smoke point and is low in saturated fat.

Adding Healthy Fats to Meals

Salads: Drizzle olive oil or avocado oil over salads. Add slices of avocado or a handful of nuts for extra healthy fats.

Smoothies: Add a tablespoon of flaxseed oil or a handful of chia seeds to your smoothie for an omega-3 boost.

Baking: Use avocado oil or coconut oil as a healthier alternative to butter or margarine in baking recipes.

Stir-Fries: Use a small amount of sesame oil or peanut oil for flavor and a healthy fat boost.

Snacks: Snack on a handful of nuts or seeds, or spread nut butter on apple slices for a healthy, satisfying snack.

Cooking Methods

Roasting: Toss vegetables in a little olive oil before roasting to enhance their flavor and add healthy fats.
Grilling: Brush meats and vegetables with avocado oil or olive oil before grilling to prevent sticking and add a delicious flavor.
Sautéing: Use olive oil or avocado oil for sautéing vegetables, meats, or tofu.
Baking: Substitute unhealthy fats like butter with healthier options like coconut oil or avocado oil in baking recipes.

Healthy fats are an essential part of a balanced diet. By understanding the different types of fats and their effects on health, you can make informed choices about which fats to include in your diet. Focus on incorporating beneficial fats, such as those rich in omega-3 and omega-6 fatty acids, while limiting harmful fats like trans fats and excessive saturated fats.

Cooking with healthy fats can enhance the flavor and nutritional value of your meals. Choose the right oils for your cooking methods, add healthy fats to your meals, and use healthier cooking techniques to support your overall health. Remember, the key to a healthy diet is balance and variety, so enjoy a wide range of foods that provide the essential nutrients your body needs.

By making small, sustainable changes to your diet and cooking habits, you can enjoy the benefits of healthy fats and improve your overall well-being.

Chapter 6: Choosing the Right Proteins

Proteins are essential for our bodies. They help build and repair tissues, make enzymes and hormones, and support overall growth and development. However, not all proteins are created equal. Understanding the different types of proteins and their sources can help you make healthier choices. In this chapter, we will explore the concept of complete and incomplete proteins, the benefits and sources of plant-based proteins, and how to make healthier choices with animal proteins.

Protein Packages: Complete vs. Incomplete Proteins

Proteins are made up of smaller units called amino acids. There are 20 different amino acids, and our bodies can produce some of them. However, there are nine amino acids that our bodies cannot make. These are called essential amino acids, and we must get them from our diet.

Complete Proteins

Complete proteins contain all nine essential amino acids in the right amounts that our bodies need.

These proteins are usually found in animal products. Examples of complete proteins include:
Meat: Beef, pork, lamb
Poultry: Chicken, turkey
Fish and Seafood: Salmon, tuna, shrimp
Eggs: Whole eggs
Dairy Products: Milk, cheese, yogurt

Complete proteins are important for overall health, especially for muscle growth and repair. They provide all the essential amino acids that our bodies need to function properly.

Incomplete Proteins

Incomplete proteins lack one or more of the essential amino acids. These proteins are usually found in plant-based foods. Examples of incomplete proteins include:
Grains: Rice, wheat, oats
Legumes: Beans, lentils, chickpeas
Nuts and Seeds: Almonds, walnuts, sunflower seeds
Vegetables: Broccoli, spinach, kale

While incomplete proteins do not provide all the essential amino acids on their own, they can be combined with other plant-based proteins to form complete proteins. For example, combining rice and beans or hummus and pita bread can provide all the essential amino acids.

Plant-Based Proteins: Benefits and Sources

Plant-based proteins are becoming increasingly popular due to their health benefits and lower environmental impact compared to animal proteins. Including more plant-based proteins in your diet can offer several advantages.

Benefits of Plant-Based Proteins

Lower Risk of Chronic Diseases: Plant-based diets have been associated with a lower risk of heart disease, type 2 diabetes, and certain cancers. Plant proteins are often lower in saturated fats and cholesterol compared to animal proteins.

Rich in Fiber and Nutrients: Plant-based proteins come with added benefits of fiber, vitamins, minerals, and antioxidants that are important for overall health. Fiber helps with digestion and can aid in weight management.

Environmentally Friendly: Producing plant-based proteins typically requires fewer resources and generates less pollution compared to animal farming. Choosing plant-based proteins can reduce your carbon footprint.

Sources of Plant-Based Proteins

Legumes: Beans, lentils, chickpeas, and peas are excellent sources of protein. They are also high in fiber and other nutrients.

Nuts and Seeds: Almonds, walnuts, chia seeds, flaxseeds, and sunflower seeds provide protein along with healthy fats and fiber.

Whole Grains: Quinoa, brown rice, oats, and barley are good sources of protein and complex carbohydrates.

Soy Products: Tofu, tempeh, edamame, and soy milk are rich in protein and can be used in various dishes.

Vegetables: While vegetables generally contain less protein, some like spinach, broccoli, and Brussels sprouts provide a decent amount.

Incorporating a variety of these plant-based proteins into your diet can help ensure you get all the essential amino acids and other nutrients you need for good health.

Animal Proteins: Making Healthier Choices

Animal proteins are a major source of complete proteins, providing all the essential amino acids our bodies need. However, it is important to make healthier choices when it comes to animal proteins to maximize their benefits and minimize potential health risks.

Benefits of Animal Proteins

High-Quality Protein: Animal proteins are considered high-quality because they contain all the essential amino acids in the right proportions.

Rich in Micronutrients: Animal products provide essential vitamins and minerals such as vitamin B12, iron, zinc, and omega-3 fatty acids, which are important for various bodily functions.

Healthier Choices with Animal Proteins

Choose Lean Cuts: Opt for lean cuts of meat, such as skinless poultry, pork loin, and beef sirloin. These cuts are lower in saturated fats, which can help reduce the risk of heart disease.

Limit Processed Meats: Processed meats, such as sausages, hot dogs, and deli meats, often contain high levels of sodium and unhealthy fats. Limit consumption of these products to reduce the risk of chronic diseases.

Include Fish: Fish, especially fatty fish like salmon, mackerel, and sardines, are excellent sources of omega-3 fatty acids. Omega-3s are important for heart health and brain function.

Incorporate Eggs: Eggs are a versatile and affordable source of complete protein. They also provide important nutrients like choline, which is essential for brain health.

Choose Low-Fat Dairy: Opt for low-fat or fat-free dairy products, such as milk, yogurt, and cheese, to get the benefits of protein and calcium without the extra saturated fat.

Balancing Plant-Based and Animal Proteins

To create a balanced and healthy diet, it is important to incorporate both plant-based and animal proteins. This approach can help you get a wide range of nutrients while also benefiting from the unique advantages of each protein source.

Practical Tips for Balancing Proteins

Mix It Up: Combine plant-based and animal proteins in your meals. For example, add beans to a chicken salad or top your yogurt with nuts and seeds.

Meatless Days: Incorporate meatless days into your week by focusing on plant-based proteins. This can help reduce your overall intake of saturated fats and increase your consumption of fiber and other nutrients.

Portion Control: Be mindful of portion sizes, especially with animal proteins. A healthy portion of meat is about the size of a deck of cards. Balancing portion sizes can help you maintain a healthy weight and avoid overconsumption of certain nutrients.

Variety is Key: Eating a variety of protein sources ensures you get all the essential amino acids and other nutrients your body needs. Include different types of beans, nuts, seeds, whole grains, and lean meats in your diet.

Cooking with Proteins

Incorporating proteins into your meals can be both delicious and nutritious. Here are some tips for cooking with proteins to make your meals healthier and more enjoyable.

Plant-Based Protein Cooking Tips

Legumes: Cook beans and lentils in bulk and use them in salads, soups, stews, and grain bowls. They can also be mashed into spreads like hummus or used as a base for veggie burgers.

Nuts and Seeds: Toast nuts and seeds to enhance their flavor and sprinkle them on salads, yogurt, oatmeal, or use them in baking.

Whole Grains: Cook a large batch of quinoa, brown rice, or barley and use it as a base for meals throughout the week. Mix with vegetables and proteins for balanced dishes.

Soy Products: Marinate tofu or tempeh before cooking to add flavor. Grill, stir-fry, or bake them for tasty additions to meals.

Animal Protein Cooking Tips

Lean Meats: Use healthy cooking methods like grilling, baking, broiling, or steaming to prepare lean meats. Avoid frying or using heavy sauces that add extra calories and fats.

Fish: Grill, bake, or poach fish with herbs, lemon, and olive oil for a flavorful and healthy meal. Fish cooks quickly and can be a convenient protein source.

Eggs: Eggs can be prepared in many ways, such as boiled, scrambled, poached, or baked. They can be added to salads, sandwiches, or eaten on their own.

Dairy: Use low-fat or fat-free dairy products in cooking and baking. Add yogurt to smoothies, use milk in soups, and sprinkle cheese on top of dishes for added protein and flavor.

Proteins are a vital part of a healthy diet, supporting growth, repair, and overall body function. Understanding the differences between complete and incomplete proteins, as well as the benefits of plant-based and animal proteins, can help you make informed dietary choices. By balancing plant-based and animal proteins, you can enjoy a variety of nutrients and flavors while supporting your health and well-being.

Incorporating proteins into your meals can be simple and delicious. Choose a mix of lean meats, fish, eggs, dairy, beans, nuts, seeds, and whole grains to create balanced and nutritious meals. Cooking with proteins using healthy methods can enhance the taste and nutritional value of your dishes.

By making small, sustainable changes to your diet and including a variety of protein sources, you can enjoy the benefits of proteins and improve your overall health. Remember, the key to a healthy diet is balance and variety, so embrace different protein sources and enjoy the journey to better health.

Chapter 7: Fruits, Vegetables, and Disease Prevention

Eating plenty of fruits and vegetables is one of the best ways to keep yourself healthy. They are packed with essential nutrients that your body needs to function properly. This chapter will explore the benefits of fruits and vegetables, explain why whole foods are better than juices, and discuss the roles of antioxidants and phytochemicals in fighting diseases.

Power of Produce: Nutrient-Dense Fruits and Vegetables

Fruits and vegetables are some of the most nutrient-dense foods you can eat. Nutrient density refers to the amount of vitamins, minerals, and other beneficial substances relative to the number of calories. Fruits and vegetables provide a lot of nutrients without a lot of calories.

Essential Nutrients in Fruits and Vegetables
Vitamins and Minerals: Fruits and vegetables are rich in vitamins and minerals. For example, oranges

and strawberries are high in vitamin C, which helps your body heal and supports the immune system. Leafy greens like spinach and kale are rich in vitamin K, which is important for bone health and blood clotting. Bananas are a good source of potassium, which helps regulate blood pressure and muscle function.

Fiber: Fruits and vegetables are high in dietary fiber, which is essential for good digestion. Fiber helps to keep your digestive system running smoothly by adding bulk to your stool and promoting regular bowel movements. It also helps you feel full longer, which can aid in weight management.

Low in Calories: Most fruits and vegetables are low in calories, making them an excellent choice for anyone looking to maintain or lose weight. Because they are high in nutrients but low in calories, you can eat larger portions without consuming too many calories.

Hydration: Many fruits and vegetables have high water content, which helps keep you hydrated. For example, cucumbers, watermelon, and oranges are all over 90% water. Staying hydrated is crucial for overall health, as water helps with digestion, nutrient transport, and temperature regulation.

Juices vs. Whole Foods: Why Whole Fruits and Veggies Are Better

While fruit and vegetable juices can be part of a healthy diet, whole fruits and vegetables are generally better choices. Here are some reasons why:

Fiber Content

Whole Foods: Whole fruits and vegetables contain fiber, which is essential for digestion and helps you feel full. Fiber also helps to regulate blood sugar levels by slowing down the absorption of sugar into your bloodstream. Eating whole fruits and vegetables helps prevent spikes and crashes in blood sugar, which can lead to better energy levels and less hunger throughout the day.

Juices: When fruits and vegetables are juiced, most of the fiber is removed. This means you miss out on the digestive benefits of fiber and may feel hungry sooner after consuming juice. Additionally, the sugar in juice is absorbed more quickly, which can cause a rapid increase in blood sugar levels.

Nutrient Retention

Whole Foods: Whole fruits and vegetables retain more of their vitamins and minerals compared to juices. Some nutrients can be lost during the juicing process, especially if the juice is exposed to heat and light.

Juices: While juices still contain vitamins and minerals, they may not be as nutrient-dense as whole fruits and vegetables. Additionally, store-bought juices often have added sugars and preservatives, which can reduce their health benefits.

Satiety and Calorie Control

Whole Foods: Eating whole fruits and vegetables can help you feel fuller longer because of their fiber and water content. This can help with weight management by reducing overall calorie intake.

Juices: Juices are less filling than whole fruits and vegetables and can be easy to overconsume. Drinking large quantities of juice can lead to consuming more calories and sugar than intended.

Antioxidants and Phytochemicals: Their Role in Fighting Disease

Fruits and vegetables are rich in antioxidants and phytochemicals, which play crucial roles in preventing diseases and maintaining good health.

What Are Antioxidants?

Antioxidants are compounds that help protect your cells from damage caused by free radicals. Free radicals are unstable molecules that can damage cells, leading to inflammation, aging, and various diseases, including cancer and heart disease.

Common Antioxidants: Some common antioxidants found in fruits and vegetables include vitamin C, vitamin E, and beta-carotene. Foods high in antioxidants include berries, citrus fruits, tomatoes, carrots, and leafy greens.

Benefits of Antioxidants: Antioxidants help neutralize free radicals, reducing oxidative stress and inflammation in the body. This can help prevent chronic diseases and support overall health.

What Are Phytochemicals?

Phytochemicals are naturally occurring compounds found in plants. They are not essential nutrients like vitamins and minerals but have protective effects on human health.

Types of Phytochemicals: There are thousands of different phytochemicals, but some well-known ones include flavonoids, carotenoids, and polyphenols. These compounds are found in a wide variety of fruits and vegetables, each offering unique health benefits.

Benefits of Phytochemicals: Phytochemicals have been shown to reduce the risk of chronic diseases, including heart disease, cancer, and diabetes. They have anti-inflammatory, antioxidant, and immune-boosting properties.

Fruits and Vegetables Rich in Antioxidants and Phytochemicals

Berries: Blueberries, strawberries, raspberries, and blackberries are rich in antioxidants like vitamin C and anthocyanins, which have anti-inflammatory and anti-cancer properties.

Citrus Fruits: Oranges, grapefruits, lemons, and limes are high in vitamin C and flavonoids, which support immune health and reduce inflammation.

Leafy Greens: Spinach, kale, and Swiss chard are packed with antioxidants like beta-carotene and lutein, which protect eye health and reduce the risk of chronic diseases.

Tomatoes: Tomatoes are rich in lycopene, a powerful antioxidant that has been linked to a reduced risk of prostate cancer and heart disease.

Cruciferous Vegetables: Broccoli, cauliflower, Brussels sprouts, and cabbage contain sulforaphane and indoles, phytochemicals that may help protect against cancer.

Carrots and Sweet Potatoes: These vegetables are high in beta-carotene, which the body converts to vitamin A. Beta-carotene is important for vision, immune function, and skin health.

Tips for Incorporating More Fruits and Vegetables into Your Diet

Eating a variety of fruits and vegetables every day can help you reap the benefits of their nutrients, fiber, antioxidants, and phytochemicals. Here are some tips for incorporating more fruits and vegetables into your diet:

Start with Breakfast: Add fruits to your morning cereal, yogurt, or smoothie. You can also include vegetables like spinach or tomatoes in your omelet or breakfast burrito.

Snack on Fruits and Veggies: Keep fresh fruits and vegetables handy for snacking. Carrot sticks, apple slices, and berries make great snacks that are easy to grab on the go.

Add to Every Meal: Aim to include at least one serving of fruits or vegetables with every meal. Add a side salad to your lunch, include a vegetable stir-fry with dinner, or enjoy a fruit salad for dessert.

Experiment with Recipes: Try new recipes that feature fruits and vegetables as main ingredients.

Look for creative ways to incorporate them into dishes like soups, stews, casseroles, and pasta.

Use as Substitutes: Substitute fruits and vegetables for less healthy ingredients. For example, use mashed avocado instead of butter on toast, replace refined pasta with zucchini noodles, or use cauliflower rice instead of white rice.

Make It Fun: Involve your family in the process of choosing and preparing fruits and vegetables. Visit a local farmers' market together, try growing your own produce, or experiment with new and exotic fruits and vegetables.

Fruits and vegetables are essential components of a healthy diet. They provide a wealth of nutrients, fiber, antioxidants, and phytochemicals that support overall health and help prevent chronic diseases. Whole fruits and vegetables are generally better choices than juices, as they retain more nutrients and fiber, which are crucial for digestion and satiety.

By understanding the power of produce and incorporating a variety of fruits and vegetables into your daily meals, you can enjoy the numerous health benefits they offer. Remember to choose a colorful array of fruits and vegetables to ensure you get a wide range of nutrients and protective compounds.

Making small changes to your diet and focusing on whole, nutrient-dense foods can have a significant impact on your health. Embrace the power of produce and take steps toward a healthier, more vibrant life.

Chapter 8: Practical Meal Plans and Recipes

Healthy eating doesn't have to be hard or time-consuming. With some planning and preparation, you can make delicious and nutritious meals every day. This chapter will provide tips for creating balanced meals, share 100 easy and healthy recipes, and offer advice for making healthy choices when eating out or on the go.

Creating Balanced Meals: Tips for Meal Planning

Planning your meals can help you eat healthier, save time, and reduce stress. Here are some simple tips to help you create balanced meals.

Start with a Plan

Set Your Goals: Think about what you want to achieve with meal planning. Are you trying to lose weight, improve your health, or save time during busy weeks?

Make a Schedule: Plan your meals for the week, including breakfast, lunch, dinner, and snacks. Write down what you will eat each day.

Check Your Pantry: Before you make a shopping list, look at what you already have. This will help you avoid buying unnecessary items.

Balance Your Plate

Include All Food Groups: Try to include a variety of foods from all the food groups: fruits, vegetables, whole grains, lean proteins, and healthy fats.

Portion Control: Be mindful of portion sizes to avoid overeating. Use smaller plates and bowls to help control portions.

Colorful Plates: Fill your plate with a variety of colorful fruits and vegetables. The more colors you include, the more nutrients you'll get.

Prepare in Advance

Batch Cooking: Cook large batches of food that you can portion out and eat throughout the week. This works well for soups, stews, and casseroles.

Pre-Cut Veggies: Chop vegetables ahead of time so they are ready to go when you need them. Store them in airtight containers in the fridge.

Cook Once, Eat Twice: Make extra portions of dinner so you can have leftovers for lunch the next day.

100 Delicious and Easy-to-Follow Healthy Recipes

Here are some easy and healthy recipes to get you started. These recipes are designed to be simple to prepare, nutritious, and delicious.

Breakfast

Overnight Oats: Mix rolled oats with almond milk, chia seeds, and your favorite fruits. Refrigerate overnight and enjoy in the morning.

Veggie Omelet: Whisk eggs with chopped spinach, tomatoes, bell peppers, and onions. Cook in a non-stick pan until eggs are set.

Greek Yogurt Parfait: Layer Greek yogurt with fresh berries, granola, and a drizzle of honey.

Avocado Toast: Spread mashed avocado on whole grain toast. Top with a sprinkle of salt, pepper, and red pepper flakes.

Smoothie Bowl: Blend your favorite fruits with a bit of almond milk. Pour into a bowl and top with granola, nuts, and seeds.

Berry Smoothie: Blend mixed berries with Greek yogurt and a splash of almond milk.

Breakfast Burrito: Scramble eggs with black beans, tomatoes, and avocado. Wrap in a whole grain tortilla.

Chia Pudding: Mix chia seeds with almond milk and a bit of honey. Refrigerate overnight and top with fruit.

Whole Grain Pancakes: Make pancakes with whole grain flour and top with fresh fruit and a drizzle of maple syrup.

Egg Muffins: Whisk eggs with spinach, tomatoes, and cheese. Pour into a muffin tin and bake until set.

Pumpkin Smoothie: Blend pumpkin puree with banana, Greek yogurt, and a bit of cinnamon.

Breakfast Quesadilla: Fill a whole grain tortilla with scrambled eggs, cheese, and salsa. Cook until crispy.

Fruit and Nut Granola: Mix oats, nuts, and dried fruit with a bit of honey. Bake until golden.

Peanut Butter Banana Toast: Spread peanut butter on whole grain toast and top with banana slices.

Savory Oatmeal: Cook oatmeal with vegetable broth and top with a poached egg and sautéed spinach.

Cinnamon Apple Oatmeal: Cook oatmeal with apple slices and a sprinkle of cinnamon.

Breakfast Tacos: Fill small tortillas with scrambled eggs, black beans, and salsa.

Berry Chia Pudding: Mix chia seeds with almond milk and berries. Refrigerate overnight.

French Toast: Dip whole grain bread in an egg mixture and cook until golden. Top with fresh fruit.

Spinach Smoothie: Blend spinach with banana, almond milk, and a bit of honey.

Egg and Avocado Toast: Spread mashed avocado on whole grain toast and top with a poached egg.

Mango Smoothie: Blend mango with Greek yogurt and a bit of almond milk.

Peach Oatmeal: Cook oatmeal with fresh or frozen peaches.

Tomato and Basil Omelet: Whisk eggs with chopped tomatoes and basil. Cook until set.

Banana Nut Muffins: Make muffins with whole grain flour, bananas, and nuts.

Lunch

Quinoa Salad: Toss cooked quinoa with chickpeas, cucumbers, cherry tomatoes, and a lemon vinaigrette.

Turkey and Avocado Wrap: Spread hummus on a whole grain wrap, add sliced turkey, avocado, spinach, and roll up.

Lentil Soup: Simmer lentils with carrots, celery, onions, and vegetable broth until tender.

Chicken Caesar Salad: Mix romaine lettuce with grilled chicken, parmesan cheese, whole grain croutons, and a light Caesar dressing.

Veggie Stir-Fry: Sauté mixed vegetables with tofu or chicken in a light soy sauce. Serve over brown rice or quinoa.

Caprese Salad: Layer tomatoes, mozzarella, and basil. Drizzle with olive oil and balsamic vinegar.

Black Bean Soup: Simmer black beans with onions, garlic, and vegetable broth. Puree until smooth.

Chicken and Avocado Salad: Mix shredded chicken with avocado, cherry tomatoes, and a lime vinaigrette.

Spinach and Strawberry Salad: Toss spinach with sliced strawberries, feta cheese, and a balsamic vinaigrette.

Vegetable Wrap: Spread hummus on a whole grain wrap, add mixed vegetables and roll up.

Greek Salad: Toss romaine lettuce with cucumbers, tomatoes, olives, feta cheese, and a Greek dressing.

Tuna Salad: Mix canned tuna with Greek yogurt, celery, and a bit of mustard. Serve on whole grain bread.

Chicken Noodle Soup: Simmer chicken with carrots, celery, and whole grain noodles in a light broth.

Egg Salad Wrap: Mix hard-boiled eggs with Greek yogurt and a bit of mustard. Wrap in a whole grain tortilla with lettuce.

Vegetable Sushi Rolls: Fill nori sheets with rice, avocado, cucumber, and carrots. Roll up and slice.

BLT Salad: Toss romaine lettuce with tomatoes, turkey bacon, and avocado. Drizzle with a light dressing.

Veggie Burger: Make a burger patty with black beans and quinoa. Serve on a whole grain bun with lettuce and tomato.

Chicken and Rice Soup: Simmer chicken with brown rice, carrots, and celery in a light broth.

Fruit and Nut Salad: Mix mixed greens with apples, walnuts, and a balsamic vinaigrette.

Taco Salad: Mix romaine lettuce with ground turkey, black beans, and salsa. Top with a bit of cheese and avocado.

Shrimp Salad: Toss mixed greens with grilled shrimp, avocado, and a light vinaigrette.

Chicken Wrap: Fill a whole grain wrap with grilled chicken, lettuce, and a bit of ranch dressing.

Vegetable Soup: Simmer mixed vegetables with vegetable broth and spices.

Pasta Salad: Mix whole grain pasta with cherry tomatoes, olives, and feta cheese.

Hummus and Veggie Wrap: Spread hummus on a whole grain wrap and fill with mixed vegetables.

Dinner

Grilled Salmon: Marinate salmon in olive oil, lemon juice, and herbs. Grill until cooked through. Serve with steamed broccoli and brown rice.

Chicken Stir-Fry: Sauté chicken breast with mixed vegetables and a light soy sauce. Serve over quinoa or brown rice.

Vegetable Curry: Cook mixed vegetables in coconut milk and curry paste. Serve with whole grain rice.

Beef and Broccoli: Stir-fry lean beef with broccoli and a ginger-garlic sauce. Serve with brown rice or quinoa.

Stuffed Peppers: Fill bell peppers with a mixture of ground turkey, quinoa, and tomato sauce. Bake until peppers are tender.

Baked Cod: Season cod with lemon, garlic, and herbs. Bake until flaky and serve with roasted vegetables.

Chicken Fajitas: Sauté chicken with bell peppers and onions. Serve with whole grain tortillas and salsa.

Vegetable Lasagna: Layer whole grain lasagna noodles with ricotta cheese, spinach, and marinara sauce. Bake until bubbly.

Shrimp Stir-Fry: Sauté shrimp with broccoli, bell peppers, and a light soy sauce. Serve over brown rice.

Pork Tenderloin: Roast pork tenderloin with a rub of garlic, rosemary, and olive oil. Serve with mashed sweet potatoes.

Grilled Chicken Breast: Marinate chicken breast in olive oil, lemon juice, and herbs. Grill and serve with steamed vegetables.

Spaghetti Squash: Roast spaghetti squash and top with marinara sauce and a sprinkle of parmesan cheese.

Stuffed Zucchini: Hollow out zucchini and fill with a mixture of ground turkey, quinoa, and marinara sauce. Bake until tender.

Turkey Meatballs: Mix ground turkey with breadcrumbs, egg, and herbs. Form into balls and bake. Serve with whole grain pasta and marinara sauce.

Vegetable Stir-Fry with Tofu: Sauté tofu with mixed vegetables and a light soy sauce. Serve over brown rice or quinoa.

Mushroom Risotto: Cook brown rice with mushrooms and vegetable broth until creamy. Stir in a bit of parmesan cheese.

Salmon Cakes: Mix canned salmon with breadcrumbs, egg, and herbs. Form into cakes and bake.

Chicken Alfredo: Make a light Alfredo sauce with Greek yogurt and parmesan cheese. Toss with whole grain pasta and grilled chicken.

Sweet Potato Chili: Simmer sweet potatoes with black beans, tomatoes, and spices.

Roasted Vegetables: Toss mixed vegetables with olive oil and herbs. Roast until tender and golden.

Chicken and Veggie Kabobs: Skewer chicken and mixed vegetables. Grill until cooked through.

Beef Stir-Fry: Sauté lean beef with broccoli, bell peppers, and a light soy sauce. Serve over brown rice.

Vegetable Pasta: Toss whole grain pasta with sautéed vegetables and marinara sauce.

Roasted Chicken: Season chicken with herbs and roast until golden and crispy. Serve with steamed vegetables.

Eggplant Parmesan: Layer eggplant slices with marinara sauce and a bit of cheese. Bake until bubbly.

Snacks

Apple Slices with Almond Butter: Slice an apple and dip in almond butter for a quick and healthy snack.

Trail Mix: Mix nuts, seeds, and dried fruit for a homemade trail mix.

Carrot Sticks with Hummus: Dip fresh carrot sticks in hummus for a crunchy and satisfying snack.

Greek Yogurt with Honey: Drizzle a bit of honey over Greek yogurt and top with berries or nuts.

Energy Balls: Mix oats, nut butter, honey, and dark chocolate chips. Roll into balls and refrigerate.

Cucumber Slices with Hummus: Slice cucumbers and dip in hummus for a refreshing snack.

Mixed Berries: Enjoy a bowl of mixed berries for a sweet and nutritious snack.

Hard-Boiled Eggs: Keep hard-boiled eggs on hand for a quick and protein-packed snack.

Popcorn: Air-pop popcorn and sprinkle with a bit of salt for a light snack.

Almonds: A handful of almonds is a great way to curb hunger between meals.

Bell Pepper Strips with Guacamole: Slice bell peppers and dip in guacamole for a crunchy snack.

Fruit Salad: Mix your favorite fruits for a colorful and refreshing snack.

Pumpkin Seeds: Roast pumpkin seeds with a bit of olive oil and salt for a crunchy treat.

Edamame: Boil edamame and sprinkle with a bit of sea salt for a high-protein snack.

Cottage Cheese with Pineapple: Mix cottage cheese with pineapple chunks for a sweet and protein-packed snack.

Celery Sticks with Peanut Butter: Spread peanut butter on celery sticks for a crunchy snack.

Frozen Grapes: Freeze grapes for a refreshing and sweet snack.

Homemade Granola Bars: Mix oats, nuts, and honey. Press into a pan and bake.

Cherry Tomatoes: A bowl of cherry tomatoes makes a simple and nutritious snack.

Yogurt with Berries: Mix Greek yogurt with fresh berries for a sweet and tangy snack.

Sliced Peaches: Enjoy fresh or canned peaches for a sweet and juicy snack.

Peanut Butter Balls: Mix peanut butter with oats and a bit of honey. Roll into balls and refrigerate.

Tomato Slices with Mozzarella: Slice tomatoes and top with fresh mozzarella and a drizzle of balsamic vinegar.

Sliced Bell Peppers: Enjoy sliced bell peppers for a crunchy and refreshing snack.

Nut Mix: Mix your favorite nuts for a protein-packed snack.

Eating Out and On-the-Go: Making Healthy Choices Away from Home

It's possible to make healthy choices even when you're eating out or on the go. Here are some tips to help you stay on track:

Eating Out

Choose Wisely: Look for menu items that are grilled, baked, or steamed rather than fried. Avoid dishes with heavy sauces or dressings.

Portion Control: Restaurant portions are often larger than necessary. Consider sharing a dish or taking half of it home for later.

Salad First: Start your meal with a salad to fill up on veggies. Ask for dressing on the side to control the amount you use.

On-the-Go

Pack Snacks: Carry healthy snacks like nuts, fruit, or whole grain crackers to avoid unhealthy options when you're hungry.

Stay Hydrated: Drink plenty of water throughout the day. Carry a reusable water bottle with you.

Plan Ahead: If you know you'll be out for a while, pack a healthy meal or know where you can find healthy food options.

Planning and preparing balanced meals can make healthy eating easier and more enjoyable. By following these tips, you can create nutritious meals that fit your lifestyle and help you achieve your health goals. With a variety of easy and delicious recipes, you can enjoy the benefits of healthy eating without spending too much time in the kitchen. And even when you're eating out or on the go, you can make smart choices that keep you on track. Embrace the journey to better health by making small, sustainable changes to your eating habits, and enjoy the rewards of a healthier, more vibrant life.

Conclusion

Key Takeaways

Eating healthy is a lifelong journey that can improve your overall well-being and longevity. The key takeaways from this book include:

Understanding Nutrition Basics: Learn about macronutrients (carbohydrates, proteins, and fats) and micronutrients (vitamins and minerals). Knowing what your body needs can help you make better food choices.

Debunking Dietary Myths: Not all dietary guidelines are accurate. Modern research suggests a balanced intake of macronutrients and a focus on whole foods.

Weight Control and Longevity: Maintaining a healthy weight is crucial for preventing diseases and improving quality of life. Incorporate balanced meals, regular exercise, and mindful eating into your routine.

Choosing the Best Carbohydrates: Prefer whole grains over refined grains and include fiber-rich foods in your diet. Understand the glycemic index to manage blood sugar levels.

Healthy Fats: Differentiate between saturated, unsaturated, and trans fats. Include beneficial fats like omega-3 and omega-6 fatty acids in your meals.

Right Proteins: Balance your intake of complete and incomplete proteins. Incorporate both plant-based and animal proteins into your diet.

Fruits, Vegetables, and Disease Prevention: Consume a variety of nutrient-dense fruits and vegetables to fight diseases. Whole fruits and vegetables are better than juices due to their fiber content.

Practical Meal Plans and Recipes: Plan your meals to ensure they are balanced and nutritious. Utilize the provided recipes to make healthy eating easier. Make smart choices when eating out or on-the-go.

Encouraging Lifelong Healthy Eating Habits

Healthy eating is not about strict diets or deprivation. It's about making better choices that you can sustain over time. Here are some tips to help you maintain healthy eating habits for life:

Start Small: Make small changes to your diet instead of trying to overhaul everything at once. This makes it easier to stick with new habits.

Be Consistent: Consistency is key. Try to make healthy choices most of the time, but don't stress about occasional indulgences.

Stay Educated: Keep learning about nutrition and health. The more you know, the easier it will be to make informed decisions.

Listen to Your Body: Pay attention to how different foods make you feel. Eat when you're hungry and stop when you're full.

Enjoy Your Food: Find healthy foods you enjoy. Eating should be a pleasurable experience, not a chore.

Stay Active: Combine healthy eating with regular physical activity. Exercise complements a balanced diet and helps maintain a healthy weight.

Seek Support: Join a community or find a buddy to share your healthy eating journey. Support from others can make a big difference.

Healthy eating is a long-term commitment to your well-being. By making small, manageable changes and staying consistent, you can enjoy the benefits of a healthier lifestyle.

Appendix

References

Here is a list of references used throughout the book. These sources provide additional information and support the content discussed in each chapter.

Harvard T.H. *Chan School of Public Health.* (n.d.). The Nutrition Source.

Mayo Clinic. (2021). *Nutrition and Healthy Eating.*

American Heart Association. (2020). *Healthy Eating.*

World Health Organization. (2018). **Healthy Diet.**

U.S. Department of Agriculture. (2020). *Dietary Guidelines for Americans*, 2020-2025.

National Institutes of Health. (2020). *Nutrition.*

Glossary of Terms

Amino Acids: Building blocks of proteins. There are 20 different amino acids, nine of which are essential and must be obtained from the diet.

Antioxidants: Compounds that protect cells from damage caused by free radicals. Common antioxidants include vitamins C and E.

Carbohydrates: One of the three macronutrients. They provide energy and are found in foods like grains, fruits, and vegetables.

Fiber: A type of carbohydrate that the body cannot digest. It helps with digestion and keeps you feeling full.

Glycemic Index: A scale that ranks carbohydrate-containing foods by how much they raise blood sugar levels.

Healthy Fats: Fats that are beneficial for health, such as monounsaturated and polyunsaturated fats. Found in foods like avocados, nuts, and olive oil.

Macronutrients: Nutrients needed in larger amounts, including carbohydrates, proteins, and fats.

Micronutrients: Nutrients needed in smaller amounts, including vitamins and minerals.

Phytochemicals: Natural compounds found in plants that have protective effects on human health.

Protein: One of the three macronutrients. It helps build and repair tissues and is found in foods like meat, beans, and nuts.

Whole Grains: Grains that contain all parts of the grain kernel, including the bran, germ, and endosperm. Examples include brown rice, quinoa, and oats.

Index

The index is a list of topics covered in the book, organized alphabetically. It helps readers quickly find information on specific subjects.

A

Amino Acids

Antioxidants

Avocado Toast

B

Balanced Meals

Batch Cooking

Beef and Broccoli

C

Carbohydrates

Chia Pudding

Chicken Caesar Salad

Nuts and Seeds

O

Omega-3 Fatty Acids

Overnight Oats

P

Phytochemicals

Portion Control

Protein

Q

Quinoa Salad

R

References

Roasted Vegetables

S

Salad

Smoothies

Spinach

T

Trail Mix

Turkey and Avocado Wrap

V

Vegetables

W

Weight Management

Whole Grains

Y

Yogurt Parfait

Acknowledgments

I would like to express my gratitude to everyone who contributed to this book. Your support and encouragement have been invaluable.

Family and Friends: Thank you for your constant support and belief in me. Your encouragement kept me going through the writing process.

Colleagues and Mentors: I am grateful for your guidance and wisdom. Your insights and feedback helped shape the content of this book.

Nutrition Experts and Researchers: Thank you for your dedication to advancing the field of nutrition. Your work provided the foundation for much of the information presented in this book.

Readers: Thank you for taking the time to read this book. I hope it helps you on your journey to better health and well-being. I hope it provides you with valuable information and practical tips to help you achieve and maintain a healthy lifestyle. Remember, small changes can make a big difference. Here's to your health and well-being!

Please, if you enjoyed reading this book, send your review across. I will appreciate it so much. Blessings!